Foreword

There are many hundreds of books 'out there' on the subject of dieting and slimming - most of them focusing on Calories, Fat and Carbohydrates - and most of them ignoring the REAL issue, which is how we THINK and FEEL about food. This book has filled that gap, perfectly. This is the first self-help book of its type that actually gives you ALL the knowledge and insight you need – in order to eat healthily and lose weight, without all the usual negatives associated with dieting.

Steve's insight into the psychological forces behind body-shape dieting and weight-loss, is second to none and I imagine this book will be used as much by health-care professionals as it will by 'the man in the Street'. Read this book, follow Steve's instructions, and you cannot help but lose weight easily AND feel great doing so.

Rob Kelly

Director of the Successful Hypnotherapy Ltd
www.successfulhypnotherapy.com

Acknowledgements

I would like to thank everyone who has supported me and helped me gain the knowledge and experience required to produce the information provided in these writings.

My wonderful fiancée Michelle, my family and close friends.

The International Association of Pure Hypnoanalysts.

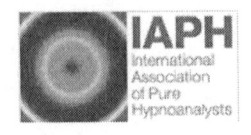

And many more. Thank you again.

Useful information

If you would like to find out about other books and future events by Steve McKeown MIAPH please see;

www.stevemckeownofficial.com

Or to book a personal appointment;

www.themckeownclinic.co.uk

Other points of interest;

www.myspace.com/stevemckeown

Slimmer Mind

By Steve McKeown D.Hyp
MIAPH

Published 2009 by Mist Publishing.
Copyright © Steve McKeown 2009

The Right of Steve McKeown to be identified as the author of this work has been asserted in accordance with sections 77 and 78 of the Copyright, Designs, and Patent Act. 1988.

A catalogue record for this book is available from the British Library.

ISBN: 978-0-9561240-0-5

All rights reserved. No part of this publication can be reproduced, stored in a retrieval system, or transmitted in any form or by any means, electronic, mechanical, photocopying, recording, or otherwise, without prior permission of the publishers.

Typeset 11/20/22 Palatino Linotype, 28/48 Willing Race

Printed and bound by Imprint Digital

Cover Design: Justin Ward Turner
Front page - Photograph by Jens Wikholm - Popstar
Website: www.popstarphoto.com
Back page - Photograph by Louise Field
Website: www.louisefieldphotography.moonfruit.com

CONTENTS

Chapter 1 16
A brief understanding of hypnosis and hypnotherapy.

Chapter 2 27
Overdoing dieting and exercise.

Chapter 3 36
A healthy way of eating, not a diet.

Chapter 4 50
Eating and exercise should be enjoyed

Chapter 5 56
Dieting and commercial diet plans.

Chapter 6 72
Understanding self-hypnosis and how it can help you lose weight and more.

Chapter 7 86
Hypnosis suggestion, formulation and application.

Chapter 8 94
How do we define what is achievable and what is not.

Chapter 9 103
Self hypnosis induction and step by step learning.

Chapter 10 119
You free MP3 download.

Chapter 11 126
Self hypnosis frequently asked questions.

Chapter 12 138
My final conclusion.

Please note:
I have included a notes page at the end of every chapter for you to add your own notes and thoughts.

A note from Steve McKeown

Welcome and thank you for taking the time to read this book. I am a member of 'the international association of pure hypnoanalysts' and have for many years been running a busy practice in St Albans, Hertfordshire. I have helped many hundreds of people, from the general public to well know celebrities, to overcome problems which affect mind and body with the use of hypnotherapy and hypnoanalysis. My in-depth specialised training has allowed me to deal with more deeply rooted problems such as depression, panic/anxiety attacks, obsessions and phobias. I have procured much experience throughout the years dealing with a variety of symptoms that any one of us could fall victim to at any time in our lives. My main focus has been working with the adverse affects which stress and anxiety have upon our bodies and minds and how they have caused everything, from the formation of habits, phobias to full blown nervous disorders.

One of the mains problems which I am confronted with

is weight issues. I have heard so many horror stories whereby people have suffered tremendously - spanning nearly all of their adult lives, either by starving themselves or by using hunger suppression remedies and simply depriving themselves.

So I have produced an easy way to lose weight. Weight gain is on the increase and I believe its not entirely your fault but society, with its constant pressure, fast pace lifestyles, fast food chains and the adverting campaigns of thousands of fad diets. So I have perfected my own healthy eating plan, with the use of self-hypnosis and believe it's one of the easiest ways to lose weight and keep the weight off, as it gives you back the control. There is no diet involved and definitely no depriving yourself in anyway.

It can be very difficult to maintain a diet or keep yourself motivated with your exercise regimes. My plan can be used to combat bad habits and help you to feel extra motivated and enthusiastic to choose healthy foods and exercise more. You really can use your mind to slim your body!

By combining deep relaxation, visualisation and concentration with hypnotic suggestion, you can replace bad eating habits with better feelings of pride and achievement within yourself and the way you look, so that you start to lose weight easily, naturally and effectively, without having to say all those horrible things to yourself.

You will also be able to learn simple yet incredibly effective psychological techniques, that will empower you and help you to regain control over your eating habits. These are effective techniques that you will learn in this book that will change your life immediately and positively.

So if you want motivation, energy, will-power, amazing mental and physical vibrancy and the ability to live your only life in a slim trim energy driven way, then take heed, read with enthusiasm and do yourself a massive favour by actually reading this book….and yes all of it, from start to finish! Most people who buy a book of this type just flick through the pages every now and again, never really understanding what it has to offer, but in order to get the full benefits from this book you must read it all, at least once.

Therapists top tips
Knowledge is power.

By arming yourself with the facts about a healthy lifestyle of eating, and ignoring the fad diets, you are more likely to build confidence in your abilities and achieve your weight loss goals.

An introduction

My aim in writing this book, is to make you realise that 'Diets' and 'Dieting' are actually making it hard for you to lose weight and keep the weight off. I will explain how you can re-learn a very simple method of losing weight that you have previously had programmed in your mind, but lost throughout the years and help you re-identify these aspects, and ultimately never having to go on a diet and feel those horrible feelings of failure and torment ever again.

In the first instance I will tell about diets and why they are hindering your success in weight loss. I will then give you a simple method whereby you can re-educate your body and mind so that they can begin to work together in harmony rather than in conflict. I will also teach you how to use self-hypnosis - some people may understand this as being self-hypnosis. This will aid you in your weight loss and give you a tool that you can use in every aspect of your life, which can be practised at your own pace.

I have explained the processes as simply as possible and aim these writings to everyone. Please remember that what I describe in this book has been very successful with many hundreds of clients that I have seen. Many of my previous clients could not believe <u>how easy it is</u> and have said that some of the information that I provide they had already understood previously, but also expressed that much of the information and teachings are unique and liberating.

With regards to the subject of weight and weight loss there are not many new findings or literature of a scientific nature, which are easy to understand or implement. I have collated much information through knowledge, understanding and experience that allows you to control this distressing aspect that has made many millions of peoples lives unhappy.

I have found that each and every client that I have seen, with regards to this subject, has lost their relationship with food and nearly all of them have been controlled by food to one extent or another. I will endeavour to try and re-educate everyone who reads this book in understanding how to get back what has been lost through time, due to the lack of knowing their own physical and mental responses. I know this may sound a little arrogant, but I understand that society, over the years, has confused our own natural responses through pressure of living and conforming.

We have in some ways become far more complacent as a race, due to convenience and this in turn has created and allowed us to un-learn some of our natural instincts that we possessed at birth.

I would like to thank you in advance for choosing to read through the entirety of this book and I can only have the pleasure of helping you regain something that through no fault of you own, you have unknowingly lost.

Word of Warning

Please do not perform any self hypnosis whilst driving or operating heavy machinery or if you suffer from epilepsy or clinical depression. If in doubt please contact your doctor.

Chapter 1

•

A brief understanding of hypnosis & Hypnotherapy.

In the first instance, I would like to start by introducing you to hypnosis, what it is and how it works.

Hypnosis is a natural phenomenon and is best described as "a state of relaxation and concentration, combined with heightened awareness".

So hypnosis is (rather disappointingly one might think) just a deep natural state of physical relaxation, combined with a relaxed yet focused mind.

Hypnosis is a state almost anyone can enter if they want to. You cannot be forced into hypnosis, despite what some stage performers might want you to believe. It has to be voluntary, you have to be self permitting to enter the state of hypnosis.

In fact, if you think about it, all hypnosis is really is 'self-hypnosis'. The so-called "hypnotist" is really just a normal person who has learned how to assist a person to enter the state of hypnosis, using certain vocal or other techniques. The "hypnotist" is just the catalyst that enables a person to enter the state by relaxing their body and focusing their mind, usually with the voice of the "hypnotist". The rest is suggestion.

In many ways the hypnotist becomes the bus driver of your mind. You simply climb aboard the bus and allow the hypnotist to take you from stop to stop, with your agreement to do so.

When you actually enter the state of hypnosis, you always remain completely aware of what is going on around you and can be completely oblivious to normal conscious distraction, but at the same time remain in complete control.

This then gives reason to why some people believe that they cannot be "hypnotised". They are then, implying that they cannot relax or enter a state of relaxation which is complete nonsense. The main reasons for this belief is that most people do not realise when they are actually in this state, because they don't feel any different other than being relaxed. There are many levels of "deepness" in hypnosis, you would only need to enter a fairly light state of hypnosis for hypnotherapy to be effective.

This means that you are fully aware of everything that is going on around you, if not more aware than you would normally be. You can hear the "hypnotist's" voice and afterwards you can remember everything that was said. You will feel very relaxed and almost lethargic. Your mind may wander off occasionally, the exact same feeling as when you are listening to the radio or watching the news on TV droning on about something boring.

There are many techniques that a hypnotist may use that can ascertain whether or not someone is relaxed and hypnotised. Generally the hypnotist will perform these tests before actually relaxing the subject but these methods are not always used within hypnotherapy.

When you return to your normal conscious awareness, at the end of a session, your eyes will open and you will simply feel relaxed, calm and contented. You are then fully conscious, fully awake, alert and immediately able to get on with whatever you want to.

Hypnotherapy and its uses.

Now there is no reason at all why anyone should have to put up with something that is inside of themselves, but outside their conscious control, as any form of anxiety can be released using hypnotherapy.

Generally, most emotional and psychological problems respond particularly well to Analytical Hypnotherapy. This type of therapy is based on the doctrine of cause and effect. The main object of analytical therapy is to search for and discover the original reason or cause of a particular behavioural problem, such as an anxiety, phobia, lack of confidence, fear or any type of complex. After revealing this the subject would have to face the original cause and relive that experience. This in turn, brings a permanent relief of the symptom and enlightenment gained.

This type of therapy uses hypnosis to aid the process of random recall of past events in the subject's life, which is known as free association. An emotionally important event from the past may be hidden or repressed from the conscious mind, but linked with behaviours such as phobias, anxieties, depression or other physical symptoms, such as a stuttering or stammering. By examining past events and allowing the associated emotion to be released, those patterns of behaviour, the symptoms, become unnecessary and therefore cease to be.

There are many problems that respond particularly well to hypno-analysis including phobias (claustrophobia, agoraphobia.), anxiety and panic attacks, migraine, sexual problems, severe eating disorders (anorexia, bulimia), stutters and depression.

The use of hypnosis dramatically "speeds up" the analytical process, achieving in a matter of weeks, what would normally be expected of the more conventional "1,000 hour analysis". Analytical Therapy usually takes

8 to 12 weekly sessions, of about 50 minutes each, although this is only a guideline as every person is unique and each individuals needs differ accordingly.

What is hypnosis?

Most people when asked if they have ever been hypnotised reply "No". They are mistaken, as everyone has quite frequently been in a hypnotic state without realising it. In childhood, daydreaming, which is so real to the child, the dream or imagined situation takes the place of ordinary reality, is essentially self-hypnosis. In adult life, many people still daydream occasionally and most people will have episodes of absent-mindedness, in which they are, as we say, "in a complete world of their own".

For instance, when driving down a familiar road, you may suddenly realise that you have travelled several miles without being able to remember details of that part of the journey. However, while you were driving, you were perfectly competent, adjusting to road conditions, avoiding the pavements and pedestrians, stopping at red lights and so on, and reached your destination safely. Yet you realise that you have no memory at all of the last few miles and probably cannot remember what you were thinking about during that period. Or at another time, you may be engrossed in watching TV, or your mind being occupied with some other task and someone may ask you a question and you answer them (like you normally would) realising sometime later, the answer you gave them is mentioned again, you have absolutely no recollection of it because you were in auto-pilot mode. In these two states, much the same thing has happened as occurs in hypnosis. The consciousness of the individual concerned separates into two streams, which are out of touch with each other. You are actually conscious and aware of only one line of thought and action at this time, while the rest is being done at an unconscious level. That is hypnosis!

This is also the same in hypnotherapy. You are always aware and conscious of what is going on around you and you may actually be aware of noises outside, the tightness of your shoes, the background music, but your awareness of these is somehow slightly glazed or removed, as you are concentrating much more deeply on what is being said to you.

Hypnotherapy can change what you need to change and develop what you need to develop. Suggestions, direct or indirect and other hypnotic phenomena, therapeutic interventions, are given and utilised, so you can achieve something you want, or something that will benefit you. In this hypnotic state, that acceptance goes even deeper than it would in non-hypnotic states.

The control is within you and your mind, not the therapist.

Hypnosis can allow you to control aspects of your psyche that normally you have no direct control over.

Therapists top tips

Concise motivations.

Write down your reasons for wanting to lose weight. Having clearly identified reasons helps your feeling of commitment. Try to include reasons that aren't just about appearance, for example, 'will help me feel fit enough to do more of the things of I want to do' or 'will help my back pain'. Looking back on them can also be a very useful motivator if the going gets tough.

- Confidence; feeling of being able to achieve anything
- Loads of energy
- able to fit into all my clothes
- Help in my business

Notes page:

Chapter 2

•

Over doing dieting and exercise.

I know this is a subject that may make some readers think, oh no, not exercise. Well, I'm not stressing that you exercise but merely trying to get you to understand why some of you despise it so much and give you a deeper understanding and show you a similarity between exercise and the diets that have also been so distressingly unresponsive throughout the years, trying to make you understand that any reservations that you have about exercise are only created by you through lack of understanding and perception. Remember, that it is entirely up to you whether you exercise or not, but it will help accelerate the rate at with which you lose weight. It is a scientific fact that exercising produces endorphins, that give you a positive and happy feeling, which allow you to become more determined to understand/change your body and mind.

I know, from my own experience, that exercise can be a chore and making it a routine of your everyday living can be a task to start with.

General excuses that I have used in the past, are, finding time in my daily schedule, feeling tired, over-exerting myself during my last session at the gym. These are all excuses but some of them have been created by myself because I have made exercise a chore rather than something that should be enjoyed.

I will explain - when I was training for a triathlon a few years ago, I set aside time during the afternoon whereby I went to the gym for an hour and a half. My schedule in the gym started with some core resistance work, lifting weights and working all the muscle groups for around 30 minutes. I would then start my cardio work, which consisted of 5 kilometres on the treadmill, then 20 kilometres on the bike and then a further 5 kilometres on the treadmill. At this point I was exhausted and used to leave the gym very fatigued and sleepy for the rest of the afternoon. I did this every other day until eventually I just could not exert myself anymore and just gave up the gym completely for around 3 months. I now look back and realise where and why I went wrong. Again I will explain.

Every time I went, I worked to a rigid routine. Routine can be boring, first mistake. I then started to time each and every session of my cardio work out even though I'd set a training time (not to over do it) but because I wanted to see some improvement. I kept up until eventually I was trying to beat my previous effort. I was now being controlled by having to have improvement, second mistake. My third mistake was I still attended, even though I was tired, because I felt guilty if I didn't. This had now become a recipe for disaster, physically and even more so mentally, because I then in turn stopped completely, making me feel as though it was all for nothing. Now some of you may never have been to the gym or exercised at all, but the moral to this and the underline aspect that I am trying to get you to understand is, this is no different from dieting.

I know from the many hundreds of clients that I have seen, that when you start a diet you are confirming to yourself that there are going to be some compromises, such as food intake, certain food types, certain fluids, and many more things that you will not have whilst following your strict guideline.

Did you remember my mistakes? - rigid routine, improvement, feeling guilty. Are you now seeing some similarities?

Following a diet produces the same outcome. You follow a rigid routine, attentively looking for improvement with weight loss by using the scales obsessively, and now starting to feel guilty because you ate something that was not included in your particular diet. Again, a recipe to disaster, because you start to become despondent and lose interest and create more and more interest in the foods that you are being denied. You then give up, probably losing a fair amount of weight only to put it, and more, back on again. Did you learn anything from your diet routine. Of course, NO you didn't, because the next time you read a magazine that promotes another diet you get back on the dieting trail and begin to lose the weight again and the extra amount that had been gained, because you had denied yourself for so long. I could guess that you, the reader, have been dieting nearly all of your life, or have had some control over what you eat due to not wanting to gain weight. I'm not saying that it is not okay to watch what you eat because there are so many foods that are not good for you out there - such as processed foods, fatty foods, and high sugared foods, but to just simply deny these and other food that is not in your diet plan is creating deprivation. This in turn creates cravings, then follows on to anxiety in the form of mood swings, anxiety and stress. You can now start to realise that you are being controlled by food.

This negative type of control makes each and every time that you diet much harder because you expect to lose what you lost before. Again, this expectation can create anxiety and make you feel low when you realise it's not working the way that you wanted.

Subjecting yourself to diets continuously throughout your life can be bad for your health, as you may or may not know that when you YO-YO up and down in weight, you are putting a strain on your body and this could be ruining your physical weight control mechanisms.

'If diets actually worked, then there would only be one, not hundreds'.

Remember, 'deprivation creates craving, craving creates anxiety, anxiety creates an unhealthy living'.

So why do you do it to yourself, never really learning anything and then putting all that weight back on again? Well this is why you are reading my book. I will then explain a very simple and effective method and way to live a healthy life without rigidity, guilt and anxiety.

Notes page:

Chapter 3

•

A Healthy way of eating, not a diet.

You are about to learn a simple and natural way to allow your body to lose those extra pounds in a healthy and anxiety free method. So by following this healthy way of eating you begin to let go of all those unwanted feelings. So here goes.

You eat what you like. Why?

Now this is a dream come true for any person that has ever been controlled by dieting, allowing you the freedom to make your own decisions on what to eat. The main reason for this is to remove any deprivation created by conventional diets. This will also remove any guilt that you may have when choosing foods that are not within your normal choice, that previously was dictated by diets.

If you have always eaten what you have wanted at a restaurant then this will remove any feeling of guilt after, or the next day, because within this lifestyle plan you are not having to avoid any particular foods so therefore will have no regrets (use your common sense).

Eat slower when you eat and stop before you are full. Why?

This is probably the most important factor of all, and your going to ask a big WHY? By eating slowly (I mean much slower than you normally would, maybe at half the speed) you are giving your body or physical response a chance to signal to your brain that you are nearly full. When you eat at a fast pace your body does not have the chance to identify when you are full and you are then over eating without even realising. We all remember a time when we had eaten too much, the typical being Christmas day when you start to feel bloated, swollen and most of all, tired. You may or may not know why you feel so tired. It's because your body is now trying to digest the food that has been over consumed and for a period, making you want to sleep - almost a form of self coma state, where your body now wants to shut down parts of your body, allowing this process to take place. It now begs the question of how do I identify when or just before I am full? Well I always use this example in a therapy session; think of time when you went out for a meal, or got a takeaway, maybe an Indian or a Chinese. Try to remember the anticipation and excitement you have before you tuck in, then remember your first mouthful - absolutely divine! Remember that mouthful, now keep that thought in your mind and be aware of how it makes you feel. I want you to keep being aware after all of your mouthfuls, to a point when the food is now not producing that feeling anymore. This is an early signal or response that suggests you are nearing being full.

Therapists top tips
Set realistic goals!

When making changes to your diet and exercise habits start small and set a few realistic goals. If they are realistic, you are more likely to achieve and stick with them and feel successful, which in turn boosts your self-esteem and self-confidence for ongoing success.

You should probably be looking to finish and stop eating. The food has now become mundane, there is no more excitement or tantalisation to be had.
Remember, the above is very important if you are going to eat what you want.

Now there are many reasons or excuses why you carry on consuming the food. These reasons could be, the main one, eating too fast, slow down! As I have said, above you need to give your body a chance to signal to your brain that you are nearing fullness. It cannot do this if you are eating too quickly, remember there is a long gap between your mouth and intestines whereby the food is still travelling to the stomach. Before you know it, 10/15 minutes after your meal, you feel bloated and over full and have to undo your belt or jeans button.

'This extra moment on your lips has now become a lifetime on your hips'.

The next reason might be that you are now just eating because its simply on your plate and so that you are not hungry later on. Again just stop! This extra food that is being consumed is not required and will only create body fat.

The next reason, and a very common one in many of us, is that you get a feeling of guilt because you do not want to waste the food that you have paid for. Again you need to stop! Remember the plate in front of you and the amount that is provided in the meal is not made to measure you and your intake, it is a mean average. A portion that the restaurant feels is adequate to provide. You should decide when to stop and not allow the food and plate to dictate this. The next reason could be that you feel guilty because there are starving people in the world with no food, which is correct, but this is no reason for you to clear your plate, as these people will not benefit either way, and you will not benefit the extra calories over consumed, other than satisfying the negative feeling of guilt . Again, you should not feel guilty because you decide that you are full and leave a leftover on your plate. It's not your fault that the mean average is above your personal intake. When you are cooking for yourself, you will adjust your portions but may at first waste some of the food. Again do not feel guilty, this is fine, you are beginning now to make the change.

Be aware that you may at first leave the table with a slightly hungry feeling but you will find that 10/15 minutes after your meal that you are actually adequately filled, or, if you have been over cautious at first and did not quite eat enough, at least then you have contributed to your weight loss and you will get a feeling of achievement, knowing that the next time you can eat a bit more, slowly finding that stop button in your mind.

Try not to eat your main meal after 7.00pm? WHY?

Now this question lends itself to many excuses made by many people in society nowadays.

For example.

I finish work late! I have to eat with my partner because he works late! I am too busy! My job does not allow me to! My lifestyle does not allow me to eat before 7.00pm! And many, many, many more excuses. The list is long.

These excuses should never be adopted because on one hand you are unhappy with your weight and you are desperate to lose those extra pounds but on the other hand you are making excuses and not willing to make a simple change. If this is the case, you need to take a long hard look at the lifestyle you are leading, as it is ruining your health and in actual fact it's shortening it. Things you could do to alleviate this problem are; eat your main meal at lunchtime and have a sandwich for dinner on the way home, or at work whilst working. You would actually receive a double benefit from doing this, as you are having a larger meal during the afternoon when your body is at its highest metabolic rate so will efficiently use the energy supplied, making you feel more awake during the rest of your working day. Also then you will find that you are now having your lunch time meal at dinner time, and not going to bed on a main meal. Your body is now slowing down, getting ready for a rest and sleep and is burning energy at a slower rate (slower metabolism) so actually does not require as much food. Also, those of you who do not eat breakfast because you feel that you just could not face it, or find it makes you feel unwell, either with the thought or by consumption, will actually find you will awake hungry (more will be explained about breakfast time in a few moments) Remember that your health is more important than anything else because without good health, efficiency in life is then compromised. EXCUSES! Why make excuses? All you are doing is making whatever your excuse justified. This is something you need to shrug off and realise is a negative mind process, making something that you know is not right, seem fine. So from now on, no excuses!.

Eat sufficient at breakfast time? WHY?

You must have breakfast, hence the meaning;

'BREAK THE FAST, this will then enable your body to kick start your metabolism and get your body started for the day'.

Eating breakfast will also reduce your lunchtime intake which is self explanatory. Many people make the excuse of not being able to find the time to sit down in the morning and eat their breakfast. This is easy to rectify, get up earlier! Stop the excuses.

Drink more fluid! Why?

This will aid your body and reduce dehydration and will help your body to be more efficient at losing weight. On average your body requires 2 litres of fluid and this does not include coffee and fizzy drinks.

I have included one last thing that is not something that you have to do but will help when identifying those natural responses that I keep going on about.

Drink a glass of water or fluid before any food is consumed.. Why?

Sometimes your body interprets thirst as hunger and by drinking before you eat you're narrowing down any possibilities of mistaking these two feelings. Eventually, after a couple of weeks, you will be able to identify and make the right choice between these feelings.

The above simple lifestyle change is not a compromise compared to any diet plan that you have undertaken, it should not be a chore or in anyway hard but quite refreshing. Just remember that you can eat what you want but you need to follow some simple guidelines, not like a diet that takes away your control but the reverse, you take control of a problem that has been so distressingly unresponsive to previous efforts whilst following a diet. Food does not control you, you control the food and by this you will find that you have more energy and in return more confidence in life.

Therapists top tops
Be a conscious eater.

Try to make conscious choices about what you eat, especially when tempted to overeat. For example, ask yourself, 'I can eat this if I want to, but do I really feel like it?' You can then choose to eat it (or some of it), or not, as you will have considered the consequences. Not only will it help you feel in control and achieve your goals, it will stop you feeling deprived.

Notes page:

Chapter 4

•

Exercise and eating should be enjoyed.

You should never over exercise. Remember do a little at a time. Do not set yourself too many targets, enjoyment comes first and the weight loss comes second.
Remember that this is a life changing decision, meaning that you have time to lose weight. Be patient, remember exercise can assist in weight loss but again it is not imperative to do it all the time. If you go to the gym and just do 15 minutes of exercise and 45 minutes chatting then so be it, because you just might actually go again and might find yourself doing 45 minutes exercise and 15 minutes chatting. This way you have not created any expectations of yourself, hence control issues and anxiety, and before you know it you will actually exercise and want to do it because you actually enjoy it. Remember, forcing/expecting yourself to exercise creates, control issues (guilt and many other emotions).

'Control issues creates anxiety, anxiety creates lack of exercise'.

Control Issues.

What are these control issues you may ask? This is where your mind comes into conflict with your expectations, creating guilt. We all know guilt is a hard emotion to understand and reason with because it is expressionless, unlike many other emotions that we deal with on a daily basis.

You should not feel guilt. Those who do, generally have no reason to, it is those that do not feel it, that should!

The conflict is only present when you create expectation, so I simply state that you should not expect things to happen , this way you will not be disappointed and feel either guilty or upset.

Some examples of control issues in dieting and exercise:

- Having to avoid certain foods, hence craving the denied.
- Exercising frequently and over exerting yourself.
- Choosing a particular dish at a restaurant only because your diet says so but secretly wanting something else.
- Using the scales obsessively on a daily basis expecting weight loss.
- Having a target weight that is unreasonable.
- Having to see improvements in fitness or the way you look within an unreasonable time frame.

So when losing weight, focus on the long term goal which is to be healthy and lose weight slowly until eventually you simply find a happy size and weight.

Therapists top tips
Eat regular meals.

Regular meals, starting with breakfast, help you to regulate how much you eat by stabilising blood sugar levels and allowing you to recognise natural feelings of hunger and fullness. They also stop you worrying about hunger as you will know your next meal or snack is not far away! And a healthy breakfast, is not only linked to long term weight control success, but a healthier, more nutritious diet overall.

Notes page:

Chapter 5

•

Dieting and commercial diet plans.

The early understanding of the word diet is known in 'Latin' as 'a way of living', notice that it does not say deprive yourself of certain foods.

If you think of the word "diet", what springs to mind? Restrictive meals?

'Guilt producing health fanatics, who can make you feel that anything that you want to eat is not only bad for your health but will ultimately end your life and it will be all your doing because you didn't listen to them and follow their diet, well maybe I went a little over board on that last one but you can see how things have been mis-interpreted'.

It can be somewhat hard maintaining a diet plan or keeping yourself motivated with any type of exercise regime at the same time. In fact you are tending to be controlled by the food and in most cases by the exercise too, as I explained earlier, this is then leaving you feeling over worked and exhausted and still trying to keep up those normal tasks of everyday living. I know from experience that most diets are worked out on a calorie intake and some are packaged up hiding this value. Again they may provide you with a daily value that for your size and weight, on average you can consume. We all know that every human being is different and that all of us have various/different metabolic rates so to simply have an average throughout a population would suggest that some people will go hungry and struggle more than the normal dieter that falls into that presumed average. This type of average can begin to make you realise that to follow a dieting plan that is directed to an entire population with no personalisation is never really going to be a success, but merely a hit and hope success rate. Even then, when we are successfully losing the weight, not learning anything other than how to be controlled and deprived by food, hence learning to ignore natural feelings of hunger taking them a step further away from ever being able to rid themselves of their initial torment.

You can see why you struggle with any diet plan due to the lack of understanding by its designer and promoter and that any diet plan has a value and is sold to make a profit so does not always have every dieter in mind.

'So don't be fooled by a billion pound industry'.

My point is that you already have the tool in your physical and mental make up, but society has in someway clouded this natural response and signal, due to complacency that has been created by you as I have explained several times earlier in the book. If you think about it, over time and generations, we have become lazier and less active. This is apparent as we now don't walk to work, we drive, we now don't tend to add up sums in our head, we use a calculator, we don't hand write letters having to worry about spelling mistakes because we email and do a spell check. There are many thousands of examples where in life we are becoming less and less active, even down to small things, as I described above. Now you can understand where your relationship with food has disappeared. The natural response that you are full, the amount of food we consume, not being able to identify between thirst and hunger. It is not a million miles away until we just simply believe everything we read and in turn confuses our minds, not knowing what to believe and what is correct because the human body and mind is designed to adapt to its surroundings, so therefore, we would simply lose even what we have now in a few generations time, not forgetting what have done even in the last 50 years.

Therapists top tips
Beware 'all or nothing' thinking'.

You know that feeling when you really overdo the chocolate or a night out and think you've blown it so may as well give up – and keep on eating... The blow out isn't a problem, but your reaction could be. Lapses are a normal part of change. You can't be, nor need to be perfect 100% all of the time to lose weight. Doing well 80-90% of the time is great progress. Rather than feel you have failed and give up, look at what you can learn from a bad day or week and plan to do things differently in the future. Then forgive, talk positively to yourself about what you have achieved already, and get back on track.

By reading through this book you can start to understand how you can make a difference and start to understand yourself and your natural signals and not be controlled by outside influences and start to

'Make up our own minds'.

Self-hypnosis and the simple routine that I am offering can be used to combat this forgotten natural response and then begin to help you to feel extra motivated and enthusiastic about eating healthy foods rather than being told.

We all know that if you were told you couldn't have something as a child, the more you would behave badly until you got it, this has not really changed as you have got older but we are tending to do it to ourselves.

If I said to you that 'you can never eat a chocolate bar ever again for the rest of your life', even if you don't eat chocolate bars on a regular basis or even once a year.

If you really think about it, give a minute or so, really

believe what I have said, you're not allowed ever! I guarantee, unless you just hate them. You will begin to feel deprived, you will be asking yourself, why? Why can't I have one, and slowly but surely you will desire one and the feeling will get stronger and stronger. This just proves that even insignificant things that you probably do not normally crave can create a conflict in your mind and hence give you a feeling of deprivation. Silly if you think about it, just a chocolate bar out of all the things you can eat. Now think about diets! I don't think I need to say anymore on the subject, other than most people can only last 4 weeks on a strict diet.

You will also be able to learn simple yet incredibly effective psychological techniques that will empower you and help you to regain control over your eating habits. These are effective techniques that you can put into practise immediately.

This book will give you the motivation, energy and willpower you may need to shift that extra weight and feel better about yourself. People have commented after a course of therapy that they feel happier, calmer, far more content, more relaxed and more positive than they have felt in years. They are more determined than ever to achieve their goals only because they now feel free from all the control created by dieting and no longer feel guilty when eating those nicer foods.

They can now understand they can eat what they want knowing they will not put the weight on and feel happier with no guilt issues.

Therapists top tips
Reward yourself.

If you have set yourself some specific goals, for example, to have regular meals, or lose 3lbs in 2 weeks or eat your 5 a day, reward yourself when you have achieved it, for example, with a new CD, seeing a movie, a new hairstyle, or outfit. It will also help to plan a big reward for when you have achieved your longer term weight goal. You will definitely deserve it.

From Slimmer's World to the G.I diet, from a soup diet to the latest celebrity diet - not a day, or a minute, goes by without the newest and best diet for one and all. There are also fat burning pills that promote unbelievable results.

The thing is, no matter what fabulous, sensationalised diet or pill that makes its way out, the fact remains conclusive - dieting will always have a 95% failure rate. People are aware of this before they start!

Despite the terrible failure rate, people still commit themselves, in their thousands, to the latest diet sensation that hits the media. All it takes is for one thin, pretty or handsome celebrity to say I live by this diet, and before you realise, every woman's magazine has written a detailed article on it and put it on the front cover. TV programmes are inviting members of the public to put it to the test and the likes of big stores, WH Smith and Amazon are swiftly producing new store space.

'One thing that you must all be realising all diets have in common is that none of them deal with the underline problem of the mental side of dieting, which is the exact reason why the majority of people that go on diets fail'.

We also know that some diets are destined to end in disaster because of the restriction and the little you are allowed to eat and especially the lack of good nutrition. However, the overall majority of diets never actually work, not because of physical deprivation for food, but mainly because of the feeling of mental deprivation.

Mental deprivation explained.

When a person decides to give up, or refrain from, a certain food for their diet, they can overly obsess over the particular food that they have decided not to have.

i.e. have you ever tried NOT to eat that wonderful delight in the cupboard and then eventually you just can't resist anymore, and your thoughts are consumed? Well this is the deprivation causing the cravings.

Hence the law of reversed effort.

The human mind has general rules, natural laws that govern its ways of functioning. One of the most important rules we all need to get to know is The Hypnotic Law of reversed effort.

This law simply states, that the harder you focus on something to do, the harder it becomes or even worse, For example, the harder you'll try consciously to encourage yourself not to eat that cream cake because you're on a diet, the harder it becomes to achieve your target.

Another example, the harder you try to force yourself consciously (with reason, persuasion, etc.) to sleep, the more and more awake you will be.

Reversed effect ... you give more effort but get the reversed result.

It works under the surface. You try to force a logical conclusion, like I won't think about that cake because I will get fat or I have to sleep now because otherwise I'd be late tomorrow morning, and you the force it on the part of your mind that understands it in reverse. The subconscious doesn't obey straight orders. You say I won't eat that lovely cake because I'll be fat and your subconscious is focusing on that fact, so you keep reminding yourself of that cake, then the imagination takes hold. Here's the conclusion - you can't resist anymore, you eat that cake, and as with your sleep, you simply don't get any. Very confusing?

This is where your conscious will comes into conflict with your subconscious imagination.

If you don't feel mentally deprived in anyway then you are not on a diet. If you do - you are!

What I want to get clear is that being on diet is a way of thinking, a very mental process and is not a way of eating, and is in no way physical. Yes, you change the way in which you eat, the times and much more, which is why people think its always about the food they are not having, this is just the feeling of being on any diet plan.

Why feel the deprivation?

The feeling of deprivation is self induced. This struggle is only created by us, by the thinking that we are making some sacrifice. Its only caused by being hard done by, not having what we would normally have. But what on earth is there to have created this deprived feeling? What have we really sacrificed, really? They either restricted our system making us feel bloated and absolutely sleepy, or they produced the most common symptom, which is FAT! So why do we get anxious about not having these foods and$ beverages? It's not even that we even enjoy the actual experience of eating these unhealthy foods, because they make us feel bad afterwards!

Notes page:

Chapter 6

•

Understanding self-hypnosis and how it can help you lose weight and more.

Self-hypnosis is a powerful tool and helps in personal development but it must be used correctly. The points and tips provided in this section can help you get off to a good start and avoid many common problems associated with self hypnosis.

Why practise?

The term "practise" is commonly used when referring to doing self-hypnosis. "Practise" correctly implies a never-ending process, one in which you continually get better the more you do it; self-hypnosis is a accumulative so therefore builds every time you practise.

"Practise" is also easier to say than something like "hypnosis." "Don't bother me for a while, honey, "I'm going to hypnotise myself." Not very elegant. Besides, others don't need to know what you're going to do; "practise" is a nice easy term that tells others nothing unless they are in on it.

Don't be misled by the use of "practise." Some people on first hearing the term think they are going to have to practise for some indefinite period of time before they can actually do it. Not so. When you are practising, you are doing it.)

The pro's and cons.

First, there is no magic by which any of us, without effort, can in one fell swoop fix everything that is wrong with us. I know this fact can be deflating because I remember the over zealous expectations I had when I first found hypnosis. I somewhat told myself that hypnosis was going make me strong, good looking, irresistible to girls, a world-class athlete, and a genius.

It was not long before I discovered it was not going to be that easy.

So that's the bad news. However, I'm happy to say that the bad news is not nearly as bad as the good news is good.

The fact is that self-hypnosis eventually becomes everything (well, nearly everything) anyone could reasonably expect. You just have to work at it a little at a time. It has been my experience that most people will actually work pretty hard if they believe it will be worthwhile and achievable. And make no mistakes; self-hypnosis will reward you for your hard efforts. It is a great way to do anything that depends on your own efforts. For example: Quit smoking, lose weight or stopping anything that you want stop. Willpower won't work for lots of people, and using hypnosis is the best way to do it.

Improve friendships and your relations with spouse and others. Get to know people who are more interesting and exciting than you (and get away with it). Sleep better (alone and otherwise, if you know what I mean). Gain control over dreams, especially alternate reality improve career success. Self-hypnosis is great for improving your prospects in life.

Develop greater sales ability. We are all selling, in one way or another, so improvement in this skill can't hurt. Overcome shyness, stage fright and other fears. Be more creative. Like salesmanship, we could all use more creativity.

The good news is that all of these achievements are within the reach of just about everyone.

All that is required is the willingness to put in a little effort to learn the skills of self-hypnosis and how to use suggestions.

Self-hypnosis is a skill. I keep going on about this skill because I know what has become of us as people. We have come to expect instant fixes from medicine or science, instant gratification through raised credit card limits, and instant solutions from TV dramas.

This is not the way life is! Nothing worthwhile is easy; you have to make time and effort for any of your desires. Self-hypnosis is like, and just as demanding as, a musical instrument. Once you have mastered Self-hypnosis you can use it to improve your well-being, and you will make it look easy. But you will need to know that you worked at it, because like any skill it requires the development of correct techniques and perseverance. You have to do it right to get the most out of it and that comes only with practise.

The good news is that, once you begin to develop the skills of self-hypnosis, it really doesn't feel like hard work at all and it does seem to work like nothing else.

As it is with any skill, the development of self-hypnosis requires practise. An hour a day would be marvellous, if you could manage it, but some life styles do not grant this so 20 minutes a day is more realistic for most people.

I would assume that you may now be thinking, 'the longer I practise for, the better it will be'?

This is not the case, it is much better to practise more regularly, each day if possible, than to have one marathon practise once a week, please remember that it is accumulative, the more you practise the better you will become at the technique.

In other words, beyond a certain point, more time does not equate to better skill. You will only learn so much; there is only so much you can learn in a given period of time. Don't get in a rush because it won't do you any good. Two or three hours a day, for example, would be counter-productive.

The conclusion is; no controlled experiments have been conducted to test the time it takes to learn self-hypnosis. But you can be confident that it will not do you any good to spend too much time at it.

Therapists top tips
Eat without distractions.

Don't let your best efforts to control how much you eat be sabotaged by doing something else during meals. A study in the American Journal of Clinical Nutrition found that women who ate while listening to a story on the radio ate 70 calories more than women who ate with no distractions.

One thing that is certain, though, is that everyone can do it. Whether it takes an hour, a month, or even a year (rare), you will be able to use the skills of self-hypnosis. And while individual variation is relatively narrow, it does exist. That is, no two people learn at the same rate.

Children and hypnosis.

Age also has a bearing on hypnotisability. The very young and the very old do not respond well, sometimes not at all. Children between about four and nine respond well but should not be taught self-hypnosis. Do not allow any child to learn self-hypnosis or subject them to any form of hypnosis, if your child is suffering from any form of anxiety please refer them to a specialist therapist that deals with Child hypnotherapy.

Adolescents sometimes do well with self-hypnosis. It is probably a good idea to avoid teaching self-hypnosis to children, especially those who are younger, because they are almost always interested in it for all the wrong reasons. If you are a parent of a younger teenager, you may or may not be a good judge of whether or not your children can deal with it. Most parents think their children are exceptional; obviously, by definition, most children are not.

The suggestions used in self-hypnosis are a powerful force that directs the subconscious mind toward the achievement of consciously chosen goals. Suggestions must be specific, technically correct and positive and applied in the right conditions. Without properly prepared and applied suggestions, self-hypnosis does not yield very good results. Just practising self-hypnosis is helpful in dealing with stress and anxiety, and it might help a person to become closer to knowing him or herself. But if suggestions are not going to be used, some form of meditation might be more appropriate.

Hypnotic states or feeling.

'What is it like?' is one of the most commonly asked questions about the hypnosis."

Trance is a common and unfortunate term frequently associated with any kind of hypnosis. For the most part, especially in self-hypnosis. You will not be transported to some un-known world in outer space. Neither will you be likely to wander around with arms outstretched and a dazed look on your face. (Unless you look like that normally.)

The most often heard descriptions of the self-hypnotic

state are that you become relaxed, in a pleasant and a heightened state of awareness, aware but not caring, almost like being asleep but still wide awake, in control but not needing to do anything. You will not lose your self-control in anyway, nor will you do anything in a self-hypnotic state that you would not otherwise do, you will always be in control of your morality.

If the word 'trance' conjures up images of a coma-like state in which you lose all consciousness and are completely unaware of what you are doing, this is so far from the truth! The probability that you will have that kind of an experience in self-hypnosis is nil. Seriously, the most common description of a good self-hypnotic state is something to the effect that you are awake, but you don't care.

Remember self-hypnosis is natural phenomenon. You have experienced it countless times. When, you may ask? For example, when you are driving your car to work? There you are, surrounded by distractions of all sorts, driving your car, but not thinking about what you are actually doing "driving'. How often have you driven to work and totally forgotten the journey you have just taken? That kind of experience is a hypnotic one, one that comes about because you are focused. Any time you are focused like that you are in a state similar to or sometimes synonymous with hypnosis.

The processes by which hypnosis works are natural, gradual and comfortable. That's why it is so easy to think that the results of self-hypnosis would have happened anyway. This, in turn, causes many people to abandon self-hypnosis as soon as they have achieved their immediate goals. This is a common mistake and a huge one at that!

The main reason why it is a mistake is because, for one thing, it usually does not take long to revert back to the original condition. This is generally what happens: a person finds himself or herself overweight, fails to lose the weight after trying to diet one, twice or even many times.

The person is introduced to self-hypnosis, begins doing

it by the book, and loses most or all of the excess weight. At that point the person stops using self-hypnosis and gains the weight back in approximately the same amount of time it took to lose it. So then it's back to dieting. But something is not working because the weight losses are small and temporary. So the person decides maybe self-hypnosis really was the key after all and that maybe he or she should have stuck with it, which would have been much easier than going through the whole routine again.

You need to keep accurate records of your beginning points and remember that the process will seem deceptively natural. No matter what you achieve you will be tempted to take the credit all for "yourself," rather than admitting that self-hypnosis helped. Keep this in your mind, any process that is good enough to help you achieve your goals is good enough to stick with from now on.

Notes page:

Chapter 7

•

Hypnosis suggestion, formulation and application.

To make self-hypnosis work, you must use suggestion. "Suggestion" is how you spell out your goals and instruct your subconscious mind to achieve those goals. Once your subconscious is in alignment with your conscious goals, their achievement is practically guaranteed. You can get that alignment, but it does take a little effort you need to know how to formulate suggestions and how to apply them.

How Suggestion Works.

The human psyche has evolved in two parts. One is the conscious mind. That's the part you think with. The other part of the mind is the subconscious mind. This is the part that you are usually not aware of, yet it determines much, sometimes most, of what you do.

The subconscious mind works in surprising ways; for one thing, it does not know the difference between reality and fantasy or the results of our imagination which are often the same thing. This is partly because the subconscious mind is limited to deductive logic (more about this in a minute; don't let it scare you if you are not familiar with the difference between deductive and inductive logic).

The subconscious also works differently from the conscious mind because one of the really important jobs of the subconscious is to keep subconscious processes sub- or unconscious. That is, secret from the conscious mind.

First let's try to understand this business of logic. Deductive logic is the process of reasoning from the general to the specific. There isn't anything difficult about this process if you remember that deductive logic means applying what you know about a lot of things to one or just a few things that are similar.

For instance, just about every human being you've ever known or heard about was born with eyes. So when you hear that someone gave birth to a new baby, it is through deductive logic that you assume that that new baby also has eyes. (Put aside for a moment the sad case of birth defects. We are talking in general or statistical terms here.)

To make another example, consider the case of something you do not like to eat. But let's say, for the sake of argument, that you tried this certain food maybe three times in your life and every time you tried it you have hated it. If you were then to be offered this food at a dinner party, it would not be illogical of you to conclude that it will still not taste any better than your previous attempts to eat it. This is deductive logic, or deduction.

Inductive logic goes in the reverse direction. With induction you form generalities from specifics. This is the logic of science, in which you go from the specific to the general. You make a limited number of observations, and then generalise what you learn to the rest of the population.

Much of the uniqueness and contradiction that is learnt in the subconscious mind is possible because it is limited to deductive reasoning.

Why is this important in a discussion about suggestion.

Because it means that a positive suggestion repeated often enough and long enough will be accepted by the subconscious mind as true. It is this characteristic that allows us to make statements that, in the beginning, are not really true, but that eventually become true. This is basically what we do with suggestion.

Please notice that I said 'positive' suggestions. That means that if the suggestion is formulated correctly, and if it is not of a nature to cause much resistance, it will work. That is, it will become true. Or more correctly, the subconscious mind will sooner or later come to believe the statement in the suggestion.

<u>When the subconscious believes it is true, it is true.</u>

Here is a simple example. A person has trouble sleeping at night. They go to bed exhausted, fall asleep almost immediately, then wake up at, say, around two in the morning and can't get back to sleep until five or six. They are not getting enough sleep and they are exhausted when they have to get up and go to work every morning. They know (consciously) they need sleep, they are desperate to get enough sleep, yet this has been going on for some time and nothing seems to work.

Now, if it were just up to their conscious mind, they would go to sleep and stay asleep until they had to get up. But something beyond their conscious mind is waking them up, and that something is their subconscious. We don't know what it is. But unless someone else is playing dirty tricks on them, it is their subconscious mind that wants them awake every night at that time.

So they formulate a suggestion to use during self-hypnosis that goes something like this: "Every night I will go promptly to sleep and stay restfully asleep until it is time to get up in the morning." (Stating a specific time to awaken in the morning would be even better.)

It may take only one recital, one repeating, of this suggestion for it to work. But it is more likely to take a week or two of daily repetitions for the subconscious to begin to believe it. Once it does, the subconscious need to awaken in the middle of the night will have been displaced with the belief that it is better to sleep through the night.

It is important to keep in mind that many things can get in the way of the effectiveness of suggestions and keep them from being good ones. Your job is to minimise the risk of triggering one of those things, and to formulate and apply suggestions that get you where you want to go.

Notes page:

Chapter 8

•

How do we define what is achievable and what is not.

The confidentiality promise taken by a Hypnotherapist includes the statement that they will not "do any harm". That would be a good addition to anyone's thinking who is working with suggestions. Suggestions that are flawed or that go against subconscious needs (negative suggestions) can make things worse. When this happens it is usually the result of errors that belong to one of the following categories.

There are such things as "can't". It always seems a little strange to have to say this but it needs to be said: try to avoid impossibilities. You are not going to grow another limb or even change yourself by becoming ambidextrous. You are not going to change your eye colour, reverse the aging process, or get rid of 3 stone of excess weight overnight. I am using silly examples to make my point here because although hypnosis sometimes seems like magic, it is not, it's a natural phenomenon.

Trying to achieve the impossible will not physically harm you, but it does do serious damage to your subconscious acceptance of self-hypnosis and any suggestions you may be working with. After all, if you are not consciously taking this seriously, why should your subconscious?

This is a tough question to answer, for example, common sense says that a woman cannot enlarge her bust size. Yet many women claim to have done just that with self-hypnosis. (This has not been scientifically proven, but try telling that to the women that tried it and had to go out and buy a larger bras.)

Equally intriguing, perhaps even more so, are the numberless findings in formal research of a placebo effect.

Placebo effects can make things seem worse under negative conditions, but they can also be used to make things a lot better. The problem is, the use of a placebo generally requires an unwitting candidate, and that clearly is not going to happen with self-hypnosis.

To conclude my attempt to answer what is possible and what is not, you'll have to use your own sense of judgment. As a main rule, approach everything gradually and just keep progressing upwards until you have reached the limits of possibility. One characteristic of the subconscious mind is that it can be really irritating when it takes everything so literally.

This tendency toward literalness can make it almost impossible sometimes to formulate a suggestion with language. In case you have never noticed this before, language can be very sloppy at times.

I suppose, considering that words are not always the things they represent, our natural confusion is over what is sign and what is symbol. And of course we make everything worse by our over-reliance on certain clichés.

The literality of the subconscious mind is its own, by that I mean that referring to dictionaries will not help a lot because those meanings may not be the same ones held by the subconscious mind or most importantly by you.

Be very aware of this when formulating your own suggestions.

Clichés are actually another form of imprecise formulation and they can create a whole world of problems when it comes to suggestion formulation. You would think that this would not be the case; since it is what you consciously mean that should be communicated to the subconscious. Unfortunately it does not work that way.

Subconsciously we tend to take things literally and what that literality is, is determined by the subconscious part of our mind. External standards like dictionaries and other sources of meaning are not going to determine the word you are going to use. This can work both ways for the subconscious. One way is the overall meaning of a word which may have the precedent meaning; the first and enduring meaning for the subconscious. This usually happens during our younger years, whilst growing up. For instance, "wicked" meant morally bad. None of the local business people around where I lived at that time would have said that REM Group music is 'wicked', or that their new car was 'wicked'. So it's not likely that I would subconsciously interpret "wicked" as anything but morally bad.

Conversely, "wicked" is now a common word and used widely, especially by teenagers and some adults who are trying to appear 'cool' in the eyes of their children. You would be wise to avoid these terms in suggestions because they are clichés and as such is rather generalised in its meaning. That is, it manages to be bland, lacking in precision, and just generally difficult to define. This is true of almost all clichés, which is reason enough to avoid them as your suggestions.

It is primarily the literal nature of the subconscious mind that makes it important to avoid clichés when formulating suggestions. A good example-using our another cliché 'cool', but in a different sense- of what can go wrong is the case of a business woman who used self-hypnosis and suggestion to get over her fear of public speaking. She formulated the suggestion that, at her next board presentation, she would be "cool, calm and collected."

At the next presentation she was indeed cool, calm and collected. She gave one of the best presentations of her career. But she was so "cool" during her presentation that she was literally shivering during the presentation by the time she was finished, as this was the interpretation her subconscious mind was having.

When formulating your verbal suggestions, search for wordings that are explicit and specific. Avoid generality as much as possible and spell out exactly what it is you want. In the case of "cool, calm and collected," our business women from the example above could have used more specific terms and phrases of a behavioural nature. To come up with this kind of formulation you will need to ask yourself, "exactly what behaviours will I be exhibiting when I am doing what I want to do, or being what I want to be"?

All of this should also serve to point out that you cannot just speed straight into a state of hypnosis, make a couple of quick suggestions for yourself, and be fixed. It will not work this way. Like I keep making a point of.

If you could use the Emile Coué formulation (Founder of law of reversed effort): "Every day, in every way, I am getting better and better." Simply add "at everything" to the end of that formulation and you would be fixed for life. But like I said, it's not that kind of world and it's not that easy.

Notes page:

Chapter 9

•

Self hypnosis induction and step by step Learning.

Now for the self-hypnosis!

Here are easy-to-follow instructions for developing a hypnotic state in you. It feels amazingly good and the results are absolutely brilliant. And it's so easy you'll be asking yourself why someone didn't tell you about this a long time ago.

Everyone, and I mean anyone, can tap into the seemingly miraculous phenomenon of self-hypnosis. All you have to do is read through these instructions, and then try it for yourself. But before you get started, let me give you a couple of time-saving tips. First, don't try and force anything to happen.

As you follow the instructions laid out for you, it is natural to try to make something happen. Being human we just naturally want to jump in and make something do what we want. But that doesn't work as well as just letting it happen.

A large part of learning to develop self-hypnosis is learning to let the hypnotic feelings take over, rather than making it happen.

Another natural tendency that often gets in the way at first is analysing everything that happens, "watching" for some "feeling" within you. I can almost guarantee that you will do that at first, and this will inhibit your hypnotic development at the beginning.

After you've practised a few times the novelty will have worn off and you will be able to keep your mind focused on what you should be doing. And don't be too sure you "know" you have or have not been in a hypnotic state. For some of us it takes a while to recognize what is going on inside of us with hypnosis. There are lots of different ways to experience hypnosis. No two people will have exactly the same experience. In one respect, though, everyone has the same experience: the hypnotic state is always pleasant.

There are no "bad hallucinate experiences to be had" in hypnosis. Keep in mind that self-hypnosis is a skill, and that you will continue to get better at it and, as you do, it becomes ever more powerful. It's a good idea to set up a schedule of practise, allowing yourself anywhere between 20 and 60 minutes, depending on how busy you are and how much time you have to spend at it. Practise during the best part of your day if you can and at a time when you are least likely to be disturbed by others. Some people are surprised to learn that they have to stay awake when they practise self-hypnosis. Hypnosis is quite different from sleep.

One interesting approach, if you have trouble staying awake, is to use suggestion to help you from falling asleep while you practise. Most people find it best to practise lying down, in a comfortable position, with as few distractions as possible. If you are bothered by noise while you practise you can try to mask out the noise with some other source of sound. You can try stereo music in the background. Later, when you have become more practised at self-hypnosis, you will be able to practise in the middle noisy room (well, almost, anyway).

The basic sections of a hypnotic induction are relaxation, deepening, suggestion application and termination.

Relaxation.

Your first job in the hypnotic induction is to slow yourself down and get yourself relaxed. But don't try to force your mind to relax .If you get yourself physically relaxed, your mind will follow.

Relaxation is really deep relaxation. It is generally an ability that most people have either lost or never developed. Some people can do it quite easily, though. They just let go of their tensions and let every part of their body become limp and relaxed. If you are one of these people, begin your self-hypnosis practise by getting nicely relaxed. Take your time. This is not something you want to rush. The time involved for the relaxation phase of your self-hypnosis induction can vary from half an hour to just a few seconds. It is an important part of the induction and should not be slighted. As you get better and your skill increases you will recognise deeply relaxed states, and you will be able to achieve them in a surprisingly short time. But as a beginner, take your time. It will be time well spent.

Deepening procedures.

Once you have completed the relaxation phase of your self-hypnosis induction procedure, you can begin to deepen the relaxed state. At some time between the deep relaxation and the deepening procedures you will move into a hypnotic state. You probably won't know it, especially as a beginner, but it will happen sooner or later.

As a beginner one of the first hurdles you must get over is when will hypnosis to happen, change in your awareness or the way you feel that will say to you, "You're hypnotised" this will definitely get in your way if you don't clear your mind. Going into a hypnotic state is, in this respect, similar to going to sleep. If you try to catch yourself going to sleep and if you try to be aware of the precise instant in which you actually go to sleep, you are much less likely to fall sleep. Being aware of this keeps you awake. In this same way you will not know when you go into a hypnotic state, or been unaware of. Later, after you have been practising regularly for a few weeks or a month or two, you'll be much more familiar with yourself and how it feels to be hypnotised.

Does it take everyone weeks or even months to get into a good hypnotic state?

No it doesn't. Some people have an amazing experience the very first time they try it. Others might practise for several days, noticing nothing, then like a tidal wave! They have one of those great induction sessions in which they know something good happened. But if you happen not to be one of these people, don't worry about it. Just keep practising and you will eventually get there, practise makes perfect.

One of the most popular deepening procedures is the count-down technique. To use the count-down technique you simply start counting downward from, say, 20 (or 100, or whatever suits you). Adjust the countdown number to whatever feels right to you after you have practised a few times.

Imagine that you are drifting deeper with each count.

Other images and thoughts will probably intrude as you count. That's fine and it is natural. Just gently brush them aside, continuing with your counting. The speed with which you count down should be natural; not too fast, not too slow. For most people this means counting at a rate of about one count for each two or three seconds. Do it at a rate that feels comfortable and relaxed to you. Some people like to tie the count with their breathing. As they drift deeper their breathing slows down, so their counting also slows down. Don't count out loud, just think your way down the count. You want to avoid as much physical involvement and movement as possible.
There are numerous deepening techniques.

You could also visualise some grand old staircase or even be stepping down a grassy hillside into a valley below, allow your imagination to take control.

How am I able to determine my depth and level of self-hypnosis?

In general, results from suggestions are the best way to determine how deep you are going in your self-hypnosis practise. If your suggestions are producing results and you are getting results of the kind you expect, then you are achieving plenty of depth in your self-hypnotic state.

Once you have reached the end of your deepening procedure you are ready to apply suggestions.

What you should have managed to do during the relaxation and deepening procedures is increase your suggestibility. That is, you have opened up your subconscious mind, at least a little bit, to receive your suggestions.

This works because of the particular, and peculiar characteristics of the subconscious part of your mind.

The most common and easiest way to apply suggestions is to have them worked out ahead of time, properly prepared wording, and memorized. It should not be too difficult to remember them because they should be rather short and you are the one who composed them. If you have them ready and memorised, you can simply think your way through them at this point. You just talk (keeping your effort to a minimum) to yourself about what it is you want to do, be, become, whatever. Don't say "you." You are thinking to yourself, so use the first person pronoun "I." Some suggestions can be succinctly stated in a somewhat more formal sort of way, like, "I am going to gain more pride and pleasure by eating in a healthy way". Elaborated suggestions are generally wordier and more of an ad lib, "food is becoming less important to me every day and I am filling my time with more pleasurable and calming pursuits than eating. "I am gaining so much achievement and pride every time I pass on desserts and other fattening foods " and so on. Although people sometimes see immediate results from their suggestions, it is more likely to take a little time for them to kick in. So be patient. On the other hand, if you have not begun to see some results within, say, a couple of weeks, you need to change your suggestions.

Creating and wording your affirmations correctly is imperative for the success you require. Work on one goal at a time, usually over a number of sessions. Don't for example work on quitting smoking and building your confidence in the same session. Although you can use a number of affirmations in one session make sure they all relate to one chosen goal at this time. Then silently and mentally repeat them over and over, slowly and positively using as few words as possible. Be very direct as though you are giving yourself commands.

Sometimes you can create a rhythm with your breathing saying the affirmation on each exhale, almost like a mantra.

When deciding on the suggestions beforehand always state them as if they are a reality and in the present. This is very important as your unconscious mind believes exactly what it is told.

For example:

Never say, 'I want to be slim'.
Say, 'I will be a very slim person'.

You need to make sure the suggestion is clear and apparent and make sure you emphasize the positive.

For example:

Never say, 'I don't want to be fat'.
Say, 'I am confident and self assured knowing that I will lose weight'.

Releasing yourself from hypnosis.

Once you have finished applying suggestions you are through with your induction and you can finish your session.

You could just open your eyes, get up and go about your business, but that is not a good idea. You should clarify the end of every session. By doing this you provide a clear indication between the hypnotic state and your ordinary conscious awareness. A clear release also prevents your self-hypnosis practise session from turning into a nap. If you want to take a sleep, take a sleep. But don't do it in a way that sleeping becomes associated with self-hypnosis practise. If you are practising at bedtime and don't care if you go on to sleep, this is okay. But still draw the line in your mind to indicate the end of your self-hypnosis session.

To terminate the session, think to yourself that you are

going to be fully awake and alert after you count up to, say, five." One, I'm beginning to come out of it, moving toward a waking state. Two, I'm becoming more alert,

getting ready to wake up. Three, and Four and Five I'm completely awake." Something along those lines.

Notes page:

Chapter 10

•

You free MP3 download.

You will be happy to see that I have also included a free MP3 download that you can now download from my official website, please go to www.stevemckeownofficial.co.uk and you will then need to type password, **hypno123**. You will find that you will have to make a choice between three hypnotic MP3 downloads and maybe wondering why this is.

You might be thinking 'oh its just another one of those hypnotic downloads which everyone receives when they get a book like this', and yes there are many books that subscribe to this method but I have, with experience tried to make this element more personal to each reader and have produced several hypnotic MP3 downloads for you to choose from.

Therapists top tips
Believe in Yourself.

This final weight controlling tip is just as important as the tips about eating and exercise.

If things go wrong don't panic. Learning new habits takes time. Think back to when you learned to ride a bike. No-one expected you to do it the first time. You no doubt fell off a lot and needed picking up, with help along the way. Step by step you took control of that bike and learned how to keep it on course.

How you think, affects how you feel, and in turn the actions you take. Believe in yourself every day. Focus on what you want – being fitter, healthier – rather than how unfit you are. Setting realistic goals and having positive expectations will make all the difference.

Why? You may ask.

This is simple! Everyone is different and everyone's needs are different.

I work everyday with different types of personality and realise that I cannot follow the same routine on every client that walks through my door, because if I did, I would not be in business.

I am going to make a wild guess and tell you that you have probably chosen MP3 download 1.

'How would I know that'?

I could be wrong, as there is a lot to take into account when assessing someone in this way but from my experience over the years I know this to be the case.

So to answer your question in full would be boring you to sleep!

How do you use the Hypnotic MP3 download?

I am hoping that you managed to get you MP3 successfully downloaded either onto a CD or on your iPod or some other MP3 player.

The best method for you is the most convenient but most people tend to download the MP3 onto their iPod/MP3 player but if you do not have this, the alternative way would be to burn the download onto CD.

Once you have managed to sort out the above.

What to do next?

Find a quite room with no interruption for at least 30 minutes and just close your eyes and let me do the rest.

How many times should I use the download?

Just to make it clear, the download that you have chosen has been produced using very effective suggestions of which I have worked on over the years to create a perfected format for weight control BUT I still suggest that you incorporate the download into your own practise of self-hypnosis.

I would suggest that for the first 14 days minimum, you try to use the download every other day if possible, also practising your self-hypnosis on the days in-between. After this time, its entirely up to you but I would like you to keep practising your self hypnosis to perfection as this will end up being a tool that will change your life in many ways as I have already explained.

Notes page:

Chapter 11

•

Self hypnosis frequently asked questions.

Is self-hypnosis safe?

It is just as safe as anything else. If you stick to self hypnosis, you have the same protective mechanisms working for you that you have any other time. You will not do anything in self hypnosis that you would not otherwise do. Of course what some people would otherwise do can surprise you.

If you have seen a stage hypnotist's show you may have seen people doing things that they would not want to do and probably would not. The only reason people do strange things in a stage presentation is because of what we call the "demand characteristics" of the situation. That is, being on stage in front of a lot of people exerts a tremendous pressure to do as one is told. It is generally wiser not to volunteer for any stage demonstrations of hypnosis, or to use it in any way just for entertainment.

Various religions in the world have at different times had something to say about hypnosis. The ancient Egyptians thought it was a Good Thing. On the other side of the coin, the Church of Latter Day Saints thinks otherwise. Some of the Church Elders believe that hypnosis is dangerous because it opens up the mind for the devil to enter. Which to be quite honest is a matter of opinion and belief.

'You can learn more about yourself when you begin to practise self hypnosis'.

What if you discover something you didn't want to know?

You can sometimes make yourself uncomfortable, but you will not hurt or create any serious problems for yourself. I have never seen a single case in which the emergence of repressed memories caused anything worse than temporary discomfort.

Self hypnosis does sometimes help a person become

more aware of his problems. But this enlightenment should not be confused with causation (which, in such a case, is a matter of blaming the messenger for the message).

Will the regular practise of self hypnosis make me more suggestible?

Yes, but only in the good sense. That is, with practise, you get better at responding to your own suggestions. This is a Good Thing because it gives you more control over yourself. At the same time, you become more resistant to the manipulative attempts of others. There is an inverse relationship between responsiveness to hetero-suggestion (suggestion applied by others) and autosuggestion (self-applied suggestion). The better you get at self suggestion, and the more you understand it and how it works, the more you become resistant to manipulative attempts by others. The regular practise of self hypnosis is great for developing discipline in those who find it difficult to "just say no."

Will you lose consciousness when you practise self hypnosis?

Only if you fall asleep. However, you might have certain areas of memory lapse later which make it seem like you were unconscious, but you were not. It is a little like the experience we have all had of doing something like driving a familiar route, only to realize later that we don't remember doing it.

What if I can't wake up?

Never happens. Getting out of hypnosis is never a problem. You'll put all of your efforts into getting into a hypnotic state, not getting out of it. The worst that can happen is that you drift off into normal sleep, in which case you will wake up, or oversleep just as you would any other time.

Everyone can learn to use self hypnosis, and how easy is it?

Yes, seemingly everyone can use self hypnosis. At least, everyone with anything approaching normal intelligence and who is conscious at least some of the time. Some people are better or faster at it than others, as is true with any skill. Regardless of where you fall on the skill continuum, you will see progress if you use self hypnosis correctly and regularly.

As to the part about self hypnosis being easy, the answer is both yes and no. It is relatively easy. That's because, as with any skill, it requires know-how and practise to develop. There is no free lunch, and you should be highly suspicious of any claims that something worthwhile is going to be easy and effortless. Self hypnosis does require some effort because it is a skill and the more you put into it the more you get out. But it is still a heck of a lot easier and faster than trying to do anything with willpower.

Are meditation and hypnosis different?

Yes. Meditative states may be similar, but the practise of hypnosis is significantly different in that it is driven by suggestion. With hypnosis there is specific work to be done.

In addition, the brain state also seems to be somewhat different between hypnosis and meditation, according to measures within science and other forms of feedback. It is not uncommon for people who do both to keep them separate, so there is obviously a subjective sense that there is a difference.

You may ask? How many things can I work on at one time with self hypnosis?

There is no answer to this question that is correct for everyone in every circumstance. It depends upon the "things" involved, how strongly the subconscious mind is attached to them, what is going on in your life at the time, and how you respond to hypnotic suggestion in general. The safest strategy for beginners is to start with just one project – perhaps an easier one – then, with some success and experience under your belt, progress to other, more difficult objectives.

You can use self hypnosis for things like relationships?

Your own behaviour, through both overtly observable and subliminal behaviours, is of paramount importance to the nature of every relationship. This includes romantic as well as career and professional relationships. And, while there is no universally accepted evidence that our minds can directly control the thoughts and behaviour of others, self hypnosis can help you control your own thinking and behaving, as well as the subliminal cues you transmit to others. In other words, yes, you can use self hypnosis to influence the behaviour of others just as if you had direct access to their thoughts (always be suspicious of the word, "control").

You can also improve your sports performance with self hypnosis?

It goes without saying that there is a strong link between thinking and sports performance. Even amateurs of any sport are acquainted with concepts like their "mental game." Self hypnosis has been shown to be influential in all forms of sports-related thinking. Many athletes use image rehearsal, a specific form of self hypnosis, to practise in their minds. This has been shown to significantly improve performance, sometimes more than actual practise.

How about pain control?

Hypnotic pain control, hypno-analgesia (controlled feeling) and hypno-anaesthesia (no feeling) – is well represented in the literature. Commonly reported are uses in dental procedures, surgical operations, and giving birth without any anaesthesia other than hypnosis. Many people have gained control over chronic pain that did not respond to any other method.

Notes page:

Chapter 12

•

My final conclusion.

Congratulations, you made it to the end, you have just learned the secret to success, never will you have to feel those horrid feelings of dieting again. Remember that this new lifestyle is not a another fad programme it really does work and this means that you will need to be patient. Give it time and you will receive the results you require.

Remember the simple guidelines that you are to follow:

- You eat what you like.

- Eat slower and stop before you are full.

- Try not to eat your evening meal after 7.00pm.

- Eat sufficient at breakfast time.

- Drink more fluid.

- Drink a glass of water or fluid before any food is consumed.

I wish you good luck and much success in your new understanding.

My offer to you.

Now that you have changed your life and have a better understanding but still feel that you would like a more practical course, why not come and see me or an associate at my clinic, where you will receive one to one therapy and support. If you do seek this route and decide to undergo therapy I will refund you the price you paid for the book.

Please also keep checking my website for other free MP3 weight control downloads and others.

www.stevemckeownofficial.com

Notes Page. (Designing your own suggestion).